I0146753

How To Be Led by the Holy Spirit: A Guide for Everyday Life

Dr. Christine Topjian (D. Min.)

Published by Christine Topjian Publishing
Toronto, Ontario
Canada
www.DrChristineTopjian.com

All rights reserved.

ISBN: 978-1-7775992-7-0
Copyright © 2022 by Dr. Christine Topjian

All rights reserved. No part of this book may be reproduced in any manner whatsoever without written permission except in the case of brief quotations embodied in critical articles and reviews.

First Printing, 2022

I wish to acknowledge the Lord and the Holy Spirit for not only giving me the idea for this book but for also providing me with the words and the images, which I hope will bless and help all who pick up this book.

I wish to also thank Carla Attardi (née Estifan) for showing me all the beauty that is available in a relationship with the Lord and how to be guided by the Holy Spirit. Your guidance started off my amazing journey.

HOW TO BE LED BY THE HOLY SPIRIT

How To Be Led by the Holy Spirit

BY AWARD-WINNING AUTHOR DR. CHRISTINE TOPJIAN

Christine Topjian Publishing

Contents

Intro

Intro

The question I am asked the most often is: "How do I hear from the Lord and how am I supposed to be led by the Holy Spirit? Is it a feeling? Is it a sensation? Does He speak with audible words? Does He speak all the time or just sometimes?"

I love being asked these questions because to me, it signals the person's possible interest in beginning a relationship with God, and it signals to me that they might like to know God's will for their lives.

So the answers to the questions are: "Yes - He can speak to you with feelings, sensations, audible words and all the time and sometimes. Like when you are talking to your best friend, you get to know their voice very well. You didn't start the relationship as best friends from day 1, it is something you built up to by spending time together, getting to know each other, getting to understand each others' ways, habits and idiosyncrasies. Your relationship with God and with the Holy Spirit is no different. You spend time with Him and you will learn more and more how He works, operates, thinks and feels. Yes, God feels and incidentally, He also loves to guide. He seeks to be invited into every aspect of your life for the purposes of bettering it."

I have come to realize over and over that God knows much better than we do; He sees 360 degrees, He is Timeless, Omniscient, Omnipresent and He can see things that we simply cannot. As such, when He guides, one would be very wise to listen, to ask probing questions and to obey.

Here is to your success, dear reader!

Other Titles by Dr. Christine Topjian

* Jesus Loves You
* Love & Kindness
* Give It To God
* Hannah Can Read e-book
* It's In Transit e-book
* The Chrissie Series: Chrissie Meditates & Visualizes
* The Chrissie Series: Chrissie Goes Places
* The Chrissie Series: Chrissie Prays
* The Canadian Residential Real Estate How-To Book
* How To Be Led by the Holy Spirit: A Guide For Everyday Life

Chapter 1

Why you would want a relationship with God

Why would you even want a relationship with God? This is a good intro question because just like anyone who is going to teach you, you want to know a bit about the Teacher.

Simply put, God is the best teacher of all.

How so?

Because He :

* He loves us more than we can possibly understand
* He knows how to reach us and knows everything about us
* He can talk to us and help us 24 hours per day, 7 days a week

* If there is someone He knows you need in your life, He knows exactly how to arrange to bring that person into your life
* He knows how to meet you exactly where you are in life and to help you exactly where you are
* His love, help and guidance cover every area of life
* He provides step by step, daily (even hourly) help and advice
* When something feels too hard, we can go to Him and ask Him to help us with it and we know that He will never give us more than we can handle
* He is able to help us in ways that at the beginning of your relationship with Him, you may not be able to understand
* As He controls everything, He is able to help us in every and any way
* He wants the best for us every day (including before you began your relationship with Him)
* He sees everything and knows the true heart of everyone
* He is the One who has assigned the Holy Spirit to live within us and to help us (He knows how to get everything done)

When we talk about a relationship with God, we are talking about an active relationship where we can feel, hear, and sense Him through the promptings of the Holy Spirit, and we can also talk to Him (either out loud or just within our thoughts) about everything.

This means that He can hear our thoughts and knows everything about us, having counted every hair on our head. He knows the best about us and the worst and loves us as a whole package.

It takes some time and some trial-and-error to learn and to understand that He wills the best for us and that when He guides, He is in fact guiding us to His best for us. The part that may be difficult for some to understand or to process is that His best for you may not be what you think you want for yourself. As such, there is a lot of trust that needs to go into this relationship.

We do come to realize (for some it can be right at the onset of the relationship, while for others it can take some time) that people can guide us, such as our friends and family, but God's guidance is the best and the most sound, so we benefit the most by following His guidance.

Just like with a best friend, it can take some time to develop this trust. You start by meeting and getting to know each other and as you see that you are in-sync, you start to open up more and more. It is much the same here.

"I can't see God so to me, He doesn't exist or matter"

This is a comment I have heard many times and while I understand it, it is important for you to see that God is a Spirit and even though you can't see Him, you can feel Him, you can sense Him, and if you engage in relationship long enough, you can certainly hear Him very clearly. This is stated in Scripture when it says:

(Jeremiah 33:3) "Call to me and I will answer you, and will tell you great and hidden things that you have not known."

The following Scripture also tells us that all Scripture is the entire word of God - which means that when you read Scripture, you can get a much better sense and understanding of who God is. This is really important because knowing how a person acts and reacts in any given context and how they behaved in history helps us get a better understanding of them.

(2 Timothy 3:16-17) All Scripture is breathed out by God and profitable for teaching, for reproof, for correction, and for training in righteousness, that the man of God may be competent, equipped for every good work.

Chapter 2

What does a relationship with God look like

"What does a relationship with God look like?"

This is a fantastic question that I am asked all the time.

The relationship will evolve over time but in the beginning, it often looks a lot like just getting to know the Lord, by such things as reading the Bible and understanding who God is and hearing about or reading the testimonial of others. You may feel led to do this because you may be going through a very difficult time and you may feel you want to turn to God for help, because you sense that something is missing and you may feel that you may want that relationship with Him, because (for instance) you are reading the Bible and you are feeling that you want to know Him better, etc. Whatever your reason for wondering about this relationship, let me commend you. It takes a strong person indeed to realize that they need some help and to choose that they want to move forward with knowing God, and to accepting to be led by the Holy Spirit.

So, as I said, this often starts by reading Scripture. I want to emphasize here that it is often very helpful to pick up student versions of the Bible because if you are anything like me, you may not understand Scripture too well (I did not understand it very well at first) and so you may need a simplified version with study-like notes, explanations, help with interpretation, etc.

It also helps to write things down in a journal to record feelings, sensations, inclinations, dates, times and more. This will help you keep a record of things that you may one day look back on and realize just how helpful this was for you. One of the advantages to writing things down is that with time, memories become fuzzy and timelines become hazy. There is nothing wrong with taking a calendar and jotting things down to indicate when you received that guidance and what you believe the guidance is to help you track things.

Calling Out

Another great thing to do is to ask God to reveal Himself to you. You can do this by calling out to Him in your mind or with your heart. Remember that God can read our minds and can sense our hearts so if you prefer calling out to Him in your mind or asking Him to sense your heart's language, He will hear that, feel that, sense that and will answer. He will answer by giving you a sense of His presence, guidance and wisdom - these are so important because they will help you realize that He is there and willing (even hoping) to have a close relationship with you, guiding you to the wisest possible and best possible answers to everything you are dealing with.

Another reason I instruct about calling out within your being and not necessarily out loud is that some people are not comfortable calling out at the beginning and that's ok. We may feel a bit foolish or we may hesitate a bit, unsure of what that will look like. It is up to you how you choose to do this and you should never be made to feel pressured or foolish when you are reaching out to the Lord. He is a loving, caring, respectful God who will never put you or anyone else in a position where you will be humiliating yourself or making a fool out of yourself. That is simply not part of His personality.

Prayer

Another thing I want to make very clear is that in prayer, you can and should pour out your heart and soul. Many people leave things bottled up inside. Please be advised that you are more than welcome to call out to God and to tell Him everything you feel about anything and everything. From your work problem to relationships to finances - He wants to be involved in every area of your life and so when you pray, you are more than welcome to pour out your heart and tell Him everything. This will without a doubt help you feel better, and lighter.

Again, I want to emphasize the point above about calling out in your spirit to His Spirit so hopefully these little diagrams will be of use and of help to you.

You can pray in silence, in your spirit, while driving in your car, while waiting at an appointment, while waiting on hold for customer service, etc. The point is, however you choose to pray, the message will get across to Him.

There is no one right way to pray. Jesus demonstrates how He prayed in the Bible and we can use that as an example but if we choose to pray while sitting or lying on the couch or any other way, the main thing is: you are praying.

When and Where

Some have asked me when and where to engage in prayer. The simple answer is: anytime **and wherever you can.** You can talk to Him at 2 am, 2 pm, in your car, at home, at work, in a bathroom stall, at a party, in your kitchen, while you are running errands, when you are feeling happy, when you are feeling sad, etc. God is everywhere so talk to Him anywhere. He wants to hear from you and He is never too busy.

You can, at literally any and every point, be as close or as far from God as you would like. When you choose to engage Him in every part of your day, you can ask Him to arrange your steps, help you schedule your day, ask Him to cause everything to fall into place perfectly time-wise in your day and He will respond every time. You can also choose not to engage Him in your day and try to control everything on your own - this is not something I would advise you to do, though, because I know for myself that if I can ask Him to make my day go smoothly with everything I have to deal with versus not having my day go smoothly and having to put out fire after fire, I would much rather invite God into my day and to have things work out beautifully.

Chapter 3

Seeing, hearing, feeling and writing it down

Seeing, hearing, feeling and writing it down

All the ways that we can hear, sense and feel God are all helpful gifts to starting or continuing your relationship with Him.

Here are some of the ways you can hear from Him:

- Having a feeling about something
- Sensing that something is right and good or wrong and just not working
- Hearing His voice (a spontaneous whisper) giving you words of wisdom about something
- When He speaks to you directly in complete words (even one word) or a sentence or phrase

· When something isn't working out as you thought it would and you sense that it is Him stopping or delaying something to protect you

Example

The following is an example of a sense or feeling that I got when I first began my relationship with Him and didn't yet have the benefit of hearing more clearly or in complete sentences.

A friend of mine and I were considering taking a trip. We had thought about where we wanted to go, the means of transportation and the particulars of where to stay, what to bring, etc. We both had an unsettled feeling about it, like something wasn't right. We had managed to book everything without issue (this was prior to covid times) but instead of feeling excited, we had an uneasy sense about the whole trip. This, in hindsight, was the Holy Spirit letting us know that something was not right about our trip. While we weren't certain what could be wrong, we definitely sensed it and with each new step to actually undertaking the trip, we sensed that this was not a wise trip to take.

Together, we asked the Holy Spirit for some clarification and to show us why this was not a good trip to take and the answer came quickly and clearly: the place we had chosen to go was experiencing a political change and there was much unrest, and to add to that, the hotel we were going to go to was in actuality experiencing a bed bugs infestation in some of the rooms (which they did not tell us about even when we spoke to them on the phone). That information was not immediately available to us because they didn't tell us, but we became aware of it through the Holy Spirit and later, the hotel admitted that it would have had to cancel our reservation because it was experiencing "maintenance issues". Had we not listened and had we taken the trip, we would have found ourselves in a very bad situation and out of a fair bit of money.

Another example I can provide for you is that of a man who had come into my life as a romantic prospect. He looked great on paper and was quite handsome. He was also pretty aggressively pursuing me and calling me/texting me as well. Everyone advised me to go for it but I knew that none of the people who were encouraging me had first prayed about it or consulted with the Holy Spirit. As such, I prayed about this and asked the Holy Spirit to guide my decision-making. Specifically, I asked the Holy Spirit to take this man away from my sight if he was not the right person for me to engage with romantically. Within 1 day of my prayer, this "perfect" man stopped calling me, stopped communicating with me and stopped showing me any interest. It was as if he fell off the face of the earth completely. I still (to this day) consider myself very fortunate that he stopped contacting me and communicating with me because now (in hindsight) I know that he was definitely not the right person for me romantically.

Asking the Holy Spirit for Clarification

You can think of the Holy Spirit as your Truth Teller. Here are some Scriptural passages to help you understand the role and nature of the Holy Spirit:

(John 14:26) But the Advocate, the Holy Spirit, whom the Father will send in my name, will teach you all things and will remind you of everything I have said to you.

(2 Corinthians 13:14) May the grace of the Lord Jesus Christ, and the love of God, and the fellowship of the Holy Spirit be with you all.

The Holy Spirit being a Truth Teller and One who is at our disposal all the time is such a gift to us. He is the One who will, in fact, tell us the truth, the reality of the situation, the true heart of a person, the true context of a situation, and much more. We as humans are limited in what we can see, so we need the help of the Holy Spirit to guide us to wise decision-making and to help us with things we cannot possibly know.

Chapter 4

Asking probing questions

Asking probing questions

Just as we ask probing and inquiring questions in school and in life to find out more and to get a better sense of things, asking the Holy Spirit for more information via probing questions is not only encouraged but is necessary, not to mention available to us 24 hours a day, 7 days a week.

No matter what you are dealing with: life, love, career, relationship, finances, investments, etc., any decision you need to make first needs to be taken to God and your answer will come via the Holy Spirit.

If you cannot sleep at 3 am and you are wondering about what you should do with something, ask the Holy Spirit. Here is a suggested question format you can use:

"Holy Spirit, I am dealing with xyz and I am not sure which way to go, what decision to take. I am asking You to help me

using the wisdom of the Lord to help me decipher what would be best and which way I should go with this decision. Please help me make the right choice and give me all the details you can to help me make the wisest choice. In Jesus' name I pray. Amen."

Then, pay attention and listen. You will surely feel, sense and have a good idea of which direction to go.

Get As Much Info As Possible

In any situation, there are many givens, variables and factors. I have found that in order to access the fullest answer, we need to ask the Holy Spirit many probing questions to get the full scope of the picture. This means that we need to ask questions about what we are dealing with from all angles. Take the example of the trip I was considering taking with my friend, here are some examples of probing questions to get a better sense of directions.

1. What do You want me to know about this trip?
2. Is it Your will for me and for us to take this trip?
3. Is there a better time to take this trip or should we just scrap the trip altogether?
4. What would have happened to us if we hadn't consulted You and we had taken the trip?
5. Is it wise to plan and to undertake any trip at this time?
6. Should we be traveling together? Is it wise for us to do so or should I travel with another person or alone?
7. Where would You advise us to go and why?

8. When would you advise us to go on this trip and why then?

In Quiet

The smartest thing to do is to ask questions when you are in silence. Just as when a person is speaking to you, it is wise to listen to them at a time when things are quiet and when we have the benefit of silence and 0 (or close to 0) distractions, in order to best hear what the Holy Spirit is saying. If you are in a crowded or loud space, go to a space that is as quiet as possible and engage in your discussion with the Holy Spirit there, so that you have the best chance of hearing, feeling and sensing as clearly as possible.

Appendix

Here are some helpful tools and resources to learn more about walking with God:

Here are some helpful websites you can refer to in an effort to help you better understand God, Jesus and the Holy Spirit. I have personally used every one of these sites and can tell you they have each helped me tremendously. They are also sites I have suggested and recommended to others. Each site has a wealth of resources to help you in every area of life.

https://www.joelosteen.com/

https://www.intouchcanada.org/

https://joycemeyer.org/

https://www.bethel.com/

https://awakenchurch.com/

https://hungrygen.com/

https://www.cluonline.com/

https://garythomas.com/

https://www.krisvallotton.com/

http://paulzanepilzer.com/

Bible Passages to Help One Understand the Lord

The following are some Bible (Scripture) passages intended to be invitations for you to come to the Lord for a loving relationship:

Come to me, all who labor and are heavy laden, and I will give you rest. Take my yoke upon you, and learn from me, for I am gentle and lowly in heart, and you will find rest for your souls. For my yoke is easy, and my burden is light. (Matthew 11:28-30)

Come to me, all who labor and are heavy laden, and I will give you rest. (Matthew 11:28)

If you ask me anything in my name, I will do it. (John 14:14)

For God did not send his Son into the world to condemn the world, but in order that the world might be saved through him. (John 3:17)

Peace I leave with you; my peace I give to you. Not as the world gives do I give to you. Let not your hearts be troubled, neither let them be afraid. (John 14:27)

But God demonstrates his own love for us in this: While we were still sinners, Christ died for us. (Romans 5:8)

About the Author

Dr. Christine Topjian is a Toronto-based educator, award-winning author and wears many hats in her day-to-day life. She holds a Doctorate in Ministry from Christian Leadership University and a Masters and Bachelors in Education from Canisius College. One of her great passions is to write books of all kinds for all ages, both fiction and non-fiction, in an effort to inspire, help, guide, lead and be of service to others.

Her website is DrChristineTopjian.com.

www.ingramcontent.com/pod-product-compliance
Lightning Source LLC
Chambersburg PA
CBHW062121040426
42336CB00041B/2232

9781777599270